FACES BY PURENESS INC

# PURE

# MENTAL

# FITNESS

*Making your mind work for you*
## BY ELIZABETH TAYLOR

*Copyright © 2023 by* **Elizabeth Taylor**

All rights reserved. No part of this book may be reproduced or used in any manner without written permission of the copyright owner except for the use of quotations in a book review.

# Contents

Introduction .................................................................. 4

How Do You Flip The Switch On Your Own? ........................... 6

My Mental Fitness Bootcamp ............................................. 19

Resilience Can Be Reactive. Mental Fitness Can Be Proactive. 23

What Are Some Exercises For The Mind? ............................. 29

Mental Fitness On Steroids ................................................ 37

# Introduction

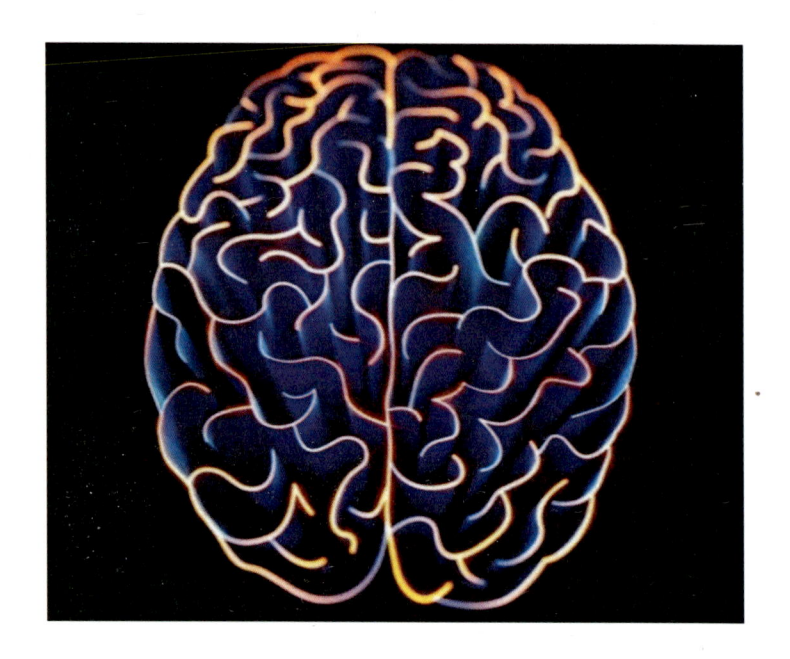

I had to organize my thoughts to propel this new journey into my career and body. It was then that everything just fell into place.

Many people start a journey to improve their health with a fantasized goal. How about changing your outlook on the goals you should set?

You will understand my point as you continue to read. This may be helpful to you, however, we are all different, and only some are suited to some approaches, including this one.

Many people think that health and fitness mean working out hard for long periods and eating undesirable foods for the rest of their lives is the only approach to long term health or natural weight loss. Consider this; you might be wrong to think this is the best way to approach your health and fitness. Perhaps change your mindset!

Look at my journey for example; it was the millionth time that I began my journey. But this time, I knew it was different. I had my mental switch on. It didn't feel like I was about to go into a boring routine for the next 12 or more months. I felt great, happy, and excited. I was mentally prepared for what was coming. Because I wasn't going to do something I hated. What I had unlocked was what I was now repeating to myself in my head.

# How Do You Flip The Switch On Your Own?

Think less. Although it sounds crazy, the first mistake is worrying too much about how difficult things will be. This can cause us to lose our way before we even begin. Worrying does not stop the problem at hand, it only adds to the existing problem. The pressure placed on the brain by worrying, doesn't help it organize your thoughts optimally. For some persons, overthinking could cause anxiety and fatigue; because not getting the job done leads to frustration. Nothing good comes out of worrying, or stressing over any particular situation. In the end it just makes you less productive, and assigned tasks, duties and responsibilities seem like an insurmountable feat.

Instead of overthinking, do it. When the flight and fight mode of the brain is activated on a daily basis, it can result in a mental condition called (ADHD) or a host of other medical complications; heart attack is also not ruled out from the list of concerns. So when you begin to worry, the first thing to do is to consider the damage that the act of unnecessary overthinking would cause to your body.

If you're already an unnecessary overthinker, then it's important you sit down, get a paper and pen, and then outline the pros and cons of that behaviour. If you carry out this exercise honestly, you will find that the cons outweigh the pros. This exercise should make it clear that there is no good reason to continue in that path that may eventually lead to several health conditions.

You need to throw the popular saying that "worrying prevents getting into a bad situation," out the window. That statement is only an excuse to support your own made up fears. The future is already unknown, and waking up with a panic attack every morning because of the fear of the future is unneeded torture.

A lot of overthinkers are so anxiety-ridden; many of them find solace in negative lifestyles as well. This in return, leads to other negative health consequences.

It's best to at least control your need to worry, and set practical steps to achieve your desired goals. With worry and overthinking out of the way, the door is open to possibilities beyond what you had ever imagined for yourself.

## Time to get started!

Eliminate foods that you know for a fact does not serve you, your body, or mind. This is ought to be the easy part; for some not so much. People tend to grow into their eating habits, and as they grow into these habits the mind forms to set plan and it becomes difficult to change if needed. For many with eating habits that hurt them, the result becomes physically evident.

Some eating habits include under or overeating, which can both include not having enough of the nutritious foods the body needs to function properly each day.

Unhealthy intake can also damage the daily health and wellbeing of an individual. It also has the possibility to reduce the life span of a person, which means the affected individuality would no longer be able to lead an enjoyable and active life.

Before permanent damage is done, assess the individual items that are missing or in excess in your diet. If you do not feel well after consuming a certain food, that can be a clear indicator that you may want to eliminate it if it is not necessary part of your daily needed intake. Missing out on or adding items to your diet that are not ideal can lead to stress, fatigue and primarily affect your ability to carry out daily activities. (You may have just unraveled the reason you are always too tired. With the passage of time, these unhealthy eating habits could contribute to the risk of developing some illnesses and other health problems.

Don't wait until your eating habits affect your wellbeing and you're in the hospital because of something you have ingested.

Let's look at this illustration; a car needs gas to move, but you decide to fill your tank with water, it would only take a while for you to have a knocked-up engine and zero movement.

When it comes to our health, the food we put in our mouth has a significant effect on all of our working parts, especially when it comes to our heart. It should not come as a surprise when you're told that too much intake of certain foods can affect the condition of your heart. Weight gain, physical inactivity, stress, high blood pressure, high cholesterol, and obesity can greatly increase the risks of heart disease and various cancers. This tells us that the heart can be affected directly and indirectly by the food we take.

When trying to quit certain eating habits, you should do more than just thinking about it, or setting unrealistic goals for the next day. Just stop immediately! Stop and don't look back. Trust me, your body will follow.

It's not about denying yourself food, but getting rid of things you know are harmful to your body right away. Trash the harmful eating habits and form great ones without a second thought. Waiting to figure out the perfect eating plan right away takes time, so this ensures that at least you are on the right path before you get the chance to overthink it and throw yourself off track.

The second important thing is that you should stop setting unrealistic goals for yourself. This is a very controversial subject. However, holding on to numbers kept me at my highest weight for so long. The idea of "I must lose 20 pounds before next month" doesn't always work. The truth is that I have learned to never set body goals, or fantasize how much weight I need to lose or when it should be done by; what clothes I want to wear or how I want them to fit. We can easily be disappointed when our goals are not met or the body does not perform as we imagined. Then we experience what I like to refer to as a 'relapse'. The disappointment makes you pick up the previous eating habits all over again, just because of a lack of first time success.

The first step to changing how you feel about your body is committing to the change. You need to be accountable to the possibility that you could be in a negative relationship with food and commit to having a real positive, healthy relationship this time around.

It is important that you learn to love yourself and your journey. Before you can learn to love your body, you need to relinquish the idea that you wouldn't feel sad, lonely, or rejected if you looked different then you wish to. As your body changes, be open to the possibilities. Be honest with yourself about what your body is capable of. You will create a healthy environment for your life and see great things happen. Unfortunately, these physical factors do affect how people treat us. This is one important lesson you have to learn on this journey. People will talk (it may be compliments or criticisms), the key thing is to be prepared. The truth is, bending over to meet people's impossible ideals and expectations will not help you feel better about yourself. The real question you need to ask yourself here is; is your body the problem, or are the worldly ideals the problem?

If you can answer the above question honestly, then you know what you want to focus your energy on. The majority opinion should not becloud your sense of reasoning.

Instead of trying to fit into a system that continually pits you against your own body, what if you adopted a new way of thinking that labels you as valuable exactly the way you are? You don't need the modifications because that's what the world perceives to be what is right or perfect.

This does not in any way validate your previous eating habits though. Do what is healthy for you, but whatever change you want to see in your body has to be because you truly want that change.

Don't clock it. Refrain from putting pressure on your body to keep working for you based upon unrealistic goals or a random finish line that you see in the future.

You may want to ask, why? Well, because not only can your body goals be unrealistic, but it can also lead to a temporary mindset. No one wants to subconsciously tell themselves that they only want to be healthy temporarily or until that special event, but that is what happens when we set certain goals within tight timelines. Setting overall goals for yourself, and then breaking them down into parts is a much more successful approach. While on a health journey of any kind we need to be kind to ourselves and be real. We may not get to where we want at exact dates, but as long as we are actively getting to the overall set goal we are still winning. What can make it very hard is seeing the journey for what it is, which is something that doesn't just end. This will help you be real with all of your inner issues and take time to heal them all. If we are being honest, trying to love your body when you really don't is not a walk in the park as the body positivity movement can sometimes make it seem.

The transition from "I hate my body" to "I love my body" does not happen easily, it takes time and intentionality.

One of the reasons why you should not set unrealistic goals like "I need to fit into my wedding dress" is that when we focus on an event or occasion as a reason for our goals, we tell ourselves that the work finished if or when we hit that goal. This doesn't mean that we shouldn't occasionally wear a suit or fit into that dress. However, it is crucial to avoid reaching your event date, then let go of all the beneficial or healthy habits you have formed. For those with a long-term goal, it would be a bit difficult sticking to a long-term journey of weight gain or loss with unsustainable plans, doing all the things you hate. This will inadvertently lead to negative thoughts and put a strain on your journey, adding to that feeling of self-doubt and making it difficult to earn the rewards you deserve.

## So what now?

That is probably the question you're asking yourself now. If you take a closer look at all that we've been discussing prior to this time, you would realize that all of the changes you're expecting to see your body, eating habits, and your reasoning starts from the mind.

The mind is the starting point of any action that is carried out by any individual. I know I mentioned earlier that you should not overthink. So you may begin to wonder, how does this work or even make sense? You can take your mind to a boot camp or perhaps even a mental fitness gym. Yes, you read those words right. You're obviously wondering how the term fitness relate with the mind.

The term fitness is often associated with the physical. The picture that comes to mind for many when this word is mentioned is someone working out in the gym or running in a park. Some dictionaries have only defined fitness to mean 'being physically fit." But fitness is beyond that, "Fitness" is a broad term that means something different to each person, but it refers to your own optimal health and overall well-being. The term overall well-being means that the body and mind are inclusive.

To function optimally as an individual, you cannot focus on the physical body and neglect your mental state. These two aspects of the human life have to be given equal attention. This is probably one of the reasons that many until recent times have neglected their mental well-being and focused on their outward appearance. Not only do you need to be physically fit, you also need to be mentally fit. You have to consider the state of your mind at all times.

While we all know we must keep fit physically, what about our mental health and well-being? We tend only to consider our mental health when there is something wrong. We don't often make an effort to improve our mental health. Majority are only concerned about their mental well-being when things fall apart, but just as sickness and diseases could be prevented, mental breakdowns can also be avoided when the mind is given the right treatment and care.

Generally, fitness is believed to be the state of health and well-being usually achieved through regular physical exercise, good nutrition and adequate sleep. Based on this definition, fitness includes everything from getting out of bed rested, eating well, exercising regularly and physically being able to survive the challenges of everyday life.

Let's paint a vivid picture; I want you to think of the mind as a storage system for everything you've experienced in life up until this moment. The reality is, this is exactly how the mind works. All that you have witnessed is entrenched somewhere in your mind, and if not resolved, it builds up into emotions that shapes our habits, viewpoints, lifestyles and actions. To live a long, psychologically healthy life which also affects our physical health, we must clear up unresolved emotional experiences. The only way this is achievable, is through mental fitness.

Clients often reach out to me as a Transformative Coach when they have a problem and need my help. People rarely make appointments because they want to stay mentally healthy. This shows that mental fitness is not seen as a proactive measure, which is one of the main causes of the high rise of mental illness we are witnessing today.

However, the transformation starts from within. As important as physical fitness is, so is mental fitness. As much as we exercise or go for walks, our mental health exercises should be just as much of a priority. Mental fitness is like physical fitness, where you're engaging in mindbody strategies, like meditation, regularly.

My only objective here is to prevent others from becoming mental couch potatoes. If you are looking for a peaceful, joyful, happy lifestyle, there are many benefits to taking care of your mental health.

Although physical fitness does not guarantee that you will never become sick, it can help to prevent future illnesses. It does put your body in the best position to handle any medical issues you may face. Mental fitness is also essential to be able to handle any mental turmoil that may come your way.

Mental fitness refers to a person's cognitive functioning and psychosocial health and well-being. You cannot address life's issues if you're not in the right frame of mind. You need to articulate your thoughts properly and be sure they are logical if you're going to be considered as a functional person. A lot of people are dysfunctional, not because they are physically healthy but because they have neglected their mental health for so long; they can no longer function properly. One thing many fail to recognize is that the mind has a great role to play in the overall well-being of the human body.

When we are mentally fit, there is a sense of positivity in our feelings, thoughts, daily habits, interactions with others and the global community. Mental fitness develops the innate ability to be emotionally healthy, which is an important part of overall health. With mental fitness you can keep your brain activities and emotional health energized and highly functional.

People who are emotionally healthy are in control of their thoughts, feelings and behaviours. It is no surprise that they cope effectively with life's challenges. Have you ever wondered why it seems like some people have it all together? My bet is that they take mental fitness seriously. Mental fitness does not mean that you will not have those emotions like everyone else, it only means that you can manage those emotions better. No one has it all figured out, they've only learned how to deal with those emotions when they come.

Emotionally healthy people still feel a spectrum of emotions, including but not limited to stress, anger and sadness. But they have developed the skills and abilities to manage their emotions, whether positive or negative, and do it effectively. One profound thing that you should note is that these individuals know how to build and maintain healthy long lasting positive connections with other people. Your emotions have a great impact on how your relationships turn out.

Mental fitness can influence how you act, think and feel, and how you choose to process stress and anxiety. Just as you train that body in the gym, you can as well train your mind. Mental fitness is an integral exercise that should be integrated into your healthy living lifestyle.

There's a tendency to define mental health by what it's not. In other words, if you don't have a mental condition then you must be mentally healthy. But that's far from the truth. That you're not suffering from a mental condition does not mean that you're mentally fit. Regardless of the unending connection of mental health to mental illness, these concepts are distinct. Mental health simply refers to a spectrum of state of our minds from low to high. Basically, if you have a mind at all, it sits somewhere on the mental health spectrum. It is your task to preserve or level up your own mental health so you can keep from experiencing breakdowns. It works the same way as your physical health, and as mentioned, mental health is distinct from mental fitness.

Mental fitness is the tool that is utilized in maintaining your mental health, just as physical fitness is needed to maintain your physical well-being. Mental health professionals like counsellors, therapists, and psychiatrists, generally treat mental health disorders and mental illness.

The goal of mental fitness is to create thought patterns and practice daily habits to help experience more positive emotions on a regular basis. If we are being honest with ourselves, focusing on negative thoughts is what eventually leads to a mental breakdown or illness. Take for example, you're having a busy day at work. Mental fitness gives you the tools to pause, stay calm and be mindful of your actions rather than let anger, stress or negative thoughts overwhelm you and potentially act out.

The ability to stay in control of your thoughts and feelings is a testament to mental fitness.

# My Mental Fitness Bootcamp

Personally, I have spent a very long time in a selfmade mental health Bootcamp. When I became a Self-Transformative Coach, my mental fitness journey began. I completed hours of speaking with others and seeing their outlooks and lives soar. So, I have continued my outward healing growth over the past several years.

Before the term 'mental health' gained popularity, I was practicing mental fitness unknowingly. I honestly did not think I had any personal or mental problems. Through my journey on the path of mental fitness, I have had firsthand experience with the countless benefits of working out from within. The hack is that it has to start from the inside – when I say 'inside' I mean the mind. It is one of the reasons I am passionate about helping others get into mental fitness.

## *Are you able to take your mindset to the gym?*
Answer: **YES**.

I know the answer to that question may seem a bit unrealistic. But if you can take your body to the gym, then why can't you take your mind to the gym. Before you took that big step to start burning calories at the gym, you had to resolve in your mind that you were going to hit the gym. The truth is, if you don't think it, you can't do it. Then it's only logical that you take care of the mind that does the thinking.

You need to also keep your brain and mental health in good shape. Including mental exercises in your daily routine (just as you hit the gym every morning) would help in shaping your mind and surprisingly, it will also positively affect your physical body. With mental fitness it is a win-win situation. If the mind is in good shape practically everything falls into place.

Mental fitness brings you to a mental state that allows you to organize your thoughts, emotions, and behaviour. This mental state is marked by well-being, resilience, and adaptability. Mental fitness, is not your entire mental health, it is however closer to stoicism, strength, or the ability to deal with the negative emotions.

There is no point denying the fact that the average human is faced with challenges each day. The question you should ask yourself is, what helps you recalibrate? When things get so tough, and you're overwhelmed, how do you manage your emotions?

This is one of the reasons why mental fitness is so essential, because it allows you to face life's challenges effectively. Mental fitness helps you to deal with stress and activates your problem-solving function. It also makes decision making easier. Mental fitness if properly utilized would help you address situations from a positive perspective and in return gives you a sense of fulfillment.

Mental fitness is more than the absence of mental illness. It's beyond self-care and recovery. It's about growth and thinking, feeling, and performing at your best in all areas of your life. Mental fitness is developed by equipping people to treat mental health as something that they can strengthen and improve.

When your body is not in the right condition, you can feel it. Two things can happen when you make this discovery; one, you decide to take a break from any functional activities, and rest. The other option is to meet a professional for diagnosis, and your doctor may ask you to take some time off to rest. But when you're experiencing anxiety, depression, or a sense of anguish, you're either oblivious or you can't place a finger on the feeling.

When it comes to our physical health, we want to be back on our feet in no time after receiving treatment which in most cases involves taking the required steps to heal. We are also exposed to the idea that even if we're no longer ill, we can increase our fitness and health to achieve a goal or level of performance. Our physical fitness can still be essential to our desired way of life.

The same can be also be applicable to our mental health. But with our mental health 'fine' is not good enough. It only means that we are not thriving, and sooner than later those negative emotions locked down somewhere in your mind would finally gain exposure. With our mental health, we don't even know the upper bounds of how truly fit we can become. Mental fitness embraces the idea that individuals can develop a positive mental state that exceeds "fine."

When you are mentally fit, you feel fully functional and confident of your ability to affect your own state of mind. It isn't that you feel "happy" all the time or that you never have an episode. The good thing about being mentally fit is that when you find yourself in that dark place, you don't fret, and you don't dwell in that place for long.

# Resilience Can Be Reactive. Mental Fitness Can Be Proactive.

B eing mentally fit can be considered taking the necessary proactive measures. Technically, your decision to be mentally fit means that you are taking practical steps to improve and maintain your mental health. Resilience, on the other hand, is reactive. Resilience is demonstrated as a result of something gone wrong, and resilience is the outcome of the fix. In simple terms, resilience can be considered a form of reactive approach or an intervention. Mental wellness can be achieved by prac ticing mental fitness.

However, the core of mental fitness is geared towards seeking potential benefits that would actually focus on enhancing mental health rather than seeking possible solutions for mental disorders or illness. When we think of the proactive approach, it is typically only met by some type of assessment or training performed in a physical sense. Why is this proactive approach not seen as a valuable ongoing routine that should be performed on our mental health?

People that are aware and mindful of their mental health are often much happier, and are more resilient than those without an awareness to proactively take care of their mental health.

Ignorance with regards to your state of mind could be a grave mistake. Mental fitness can also be used as a tool to check the state of your mind. You will discover your tendencies in the process and take the necessary steps in managing the situation.

With mental health, you should focus on prevention, not intervention. When you neglect your mental health, there is a tendency that it would result into complications in the future. It is important to integrate mental fitness in your daily routine, even when you're supposedly 'fine'. Underlying issues might seem subtle at first, but if not given proper attention they may compound over time. Anxiety is a classic example, when not managed, it could lead to other mental conditions. In some cases, patients with this condition may have to live on medications for a considerable time of their lives. As I cannot diagnose and it can be controversial to say, not all mental things need to be healed with physical medications. However, always seek the advice of your medical doctor. What is mentioned here are simply things to consider when looking at the larger scope of your mental state.

By preventing, rather than just intervening, you allow yourself to leverage your full complement of strengths and take control over the situation. You don't have to suffer a mental condition before you consider taking mental fitness seriously.

Mental fitness doesn't just provide resilience. Below are some other benefits. *Standard benefits:*

- **Greater outlook on stress and adversity:** mental fitness helps gives you a different perspective to stress and opposition. It has been mentioned repeatedly in this text that mental fitness helps you to focus on more positive thoughts rather than the negative. This does not mean that you will not experience or have these negative emotions, but it helps you put things in proper perspective.

- **Better problem-solving skills:** mental fitness also strengthens the brains muscles. This also means that the mind is capable of providing solutions when it is in the right shape. You may wonder why people need to clear their heads before they handle a serious project. Some organizations send their employees on a retreat yearly to 'cool off', all of these are done to put the mind in a position to be productive. Relaxation and meditation enhance the activities of the brain.

- **Improved decision-making skills:** For those suffering from anxiety, sometimes it is difficult to make decisions. When you're mentally fit, you're capable of organizing your thoughts and emotions. This helps with decision making especially when you need a 'clear head'.

- **Emotional Benefits:** mental fitness also helps to manage emotions. Someone struggling with emotional control may find it hard to manage strong emotions such as anger or sorrow which may lead to other complications. They may lose control over their emotions then overreact. This experience may result into mood swings, which could lead them to be overwhelmed by the intensity of their feelings. Some emotions can be overwhelming, and if not properly managed it can harmful to your well-being. Mental fitness helps with dealing with these emotions. Learning to keep your emotions in check is very important. You're at the risk of having a mental breakdown if you don't take the necessary precautions.

- **Increased self-esteem & self-confidence:** the mind could also be a place I like to refer to as 'the battleground' - the analogy is that in the mind there are a lot of conflicting thoughts. There is a constant struggle between the negative and positive thoughts. In some cases, this affects our reactions to certain situations. But with the right mindset you can focus more on the positive thought which in turn boosts your self-esteem and self-confidence.

- A more positive outlook on your life

- **Behavioural benefits:** with a positive mindset the bad and unhealthy lifestyle begins to change. Some have been subjected to substance abuse, and challenged eating habits but with mental fitness these things can be changed.

- **Increased self-control:** Research has largely shown that self-control could be a product of genetics. But several years in the journey of mental wellness field has also shown that self-control can also be developed with practice. Self-control is an important trait in the human life, as it is a set of abilities that helps an individual to plan, monitor, and achieve their goals. Even some mental conditions often have characteristics linked to problems with self-control which greatly changes their lives and overall outlook. A person who has mastered self-control is capable of exhibiting a great deal of willpower and wielding personal control. They don't act impulsively and can regulate their emotions and actions effectively.

- Improved stress management skills

- Higher resistance to temptation and healthier habits

# What Are Some Exercises For The Mind?

Now, that we have established the fact that mental fitness is important, and considered the possibility of taking our mindset to the gym; it would be pointless if we don't discuss how mental fitness works.

Mental fitness is all about reaching emotional balance, increasing awareness, making clear decisions, and setting healthy boundaries.

Mental exercises keep you mentally fit so jumping on the couch and binging watching your favourite series to "unwind" does not count as a mental exercise. You have to do the actual work.

There are different ways and types of exercises that can help in keeping your mind fit. But before we discuss the exercises that can be utilized there are certain things we need to identify.

- You need to identify the patterns or situations that trigger your emotions. When you have successfully identified these patterns, then you can find a strategy that works for you. Part of strengthening your mental fitness is discovering strategies that are most effective for you. It is different for everyone, for some meditations work while some prefer to journal.

- You also need to integrate techniques that regulate overwhelming emotions and thoughts as they surface.

- Another important thing you need to do is to resolve the patterns that detract from your well-being by building new ones. In simple terms you need to focus on building and adopting a new lifestyle.

Sometimes what you need to do is some mind-bending stretches? Well maybe not so literally, but that is basically what you are doing when you take charge of your mind. You need to conform your mind into doing the right things. The interesting thing about the mental well-being is that it has a ripple effect on your physical well-being.

Many exercises can relieve stress and help you feel calmer and more relaxed. Such as;

- Breath-work

- Yoga

- Therapy

- **Journalling:** During your mental well-being journey, journalling your process to see how far your achievements have come is ideal. Document daily. Write and keep writing. No matter how bad it sounds, it is your journal. No one is going to see it anyway. Writing down your thoughts takes the load off your mind. You begin to feel less burdened. If you don't document and record your journey, you may not see how far you have come. Which may not help you overcome your inner quest for self-awareness?

- Heart-Brain Coherence

- **Meditation:** This practice has been in existence for thousands of years. Some people postulate that meditation is older than the existence of mankind itself. No one has a precise definition of Meditation. Meditation transcends and varies from person to person. Above all, inner peace is achieved. Meditation explores mankind in several ways. When we meditate the body and mind become one. You feel a sense of calmness. If you're a yogi enthusiast, you'd notice that when you're in a state of absolute tranquility, you can listen to the rhythm of every wind movement.

Everyone wants to stay calm but certain factors distract us from attaining a meditating state. In the 17th century, a French philosopher quoted "All of humanity's problems stem from man's inability to sit quietly in a room alone." After reading this chapter, ponder on this quote. Ask yourself these questions;

- Why do I need outer noise?

- What mentally goes on in my head when silent for a while?

- What happens to my physicality when I'm quiet?

When you've answered these mindful questions then, will you begin to read more meaning to the quote above. Meditation is a personalized process. We don't function the same as humans. Even our metabolic processes differ. We don't all breathe at the same pace, and nor do we break down energy at the same time. The same applies to meditation. We get so engulfed with everyday activities that we forget to make time for our mind, and soul. We chase the worldly things we think matter, ambitions, wealth, fame, etc. Funny thing is that we think we're already making time for our minds. We think by feeding ourselves or watching that motivational video, or gathering affirmations we can find peace. Well, you're wrong. We need time for self-reflection. Just like the ancient philosophers, only you can heal yourself. No one else can, and meditation is instrumental in that healing process.

Meditation is a time for quiet reflection. Ponder on past events. It can shape your mind and soul in significant ways. Although there are events where we need to be all geared up towards being productive and energetic. Consequently, you should also make time out to relax and care for your mind.

Another aspect of Meditation is dwelling on past events. Oftentimes than not, we've heard that our past experiences shape our personalities. It influences our thought process, relations with people, and how we view life in general. Some with PTSD (Post Traumatic Stress Disorder) have this mental health obstacle that occurs as a result of negative past experiences that triggers the mind. It can cause anxiety, an increase in heart rate, migraine, and other mental syndromes.

The truth is the body knows how to heal itself. Your body is equipped with natural self-repair mechanisms.

It is only when the counterbalancing relaxation response is activated, when the sympathetic nervous system is turned off and the parasympathetic nervous system is turned on, can the body heal itself.

Meditation has been scientifically proven to activate the relaxation response, and as a result, some conditions can be greatly improved.

- Positive Affirmations (when used as an integral step and not the cure)

All of these are what I have found relevant in my journey, and when helping others they found very useful to get to a state of mental wellness. Like I mentioned earlier, you need to choose what suits you. Find what works for you then work with it. It is a gradual process, and you need to understand that the fix doesn't happen immediately. As you progress on the journey of mental fitness you will begin to experience the changes in managing your emotions.

Mental Fitness also delivers a host of benefits. It equally creates an environment where people feel less pressured, less stressed and less isolated. It provides the necessary tools to address issues in non-confrontational ways (wave of emotions) to handle life's hiccups. One of the profound things that mental fitness does is that it opens a communication link between people that are in a moment of strong feelings. It creates a platform where people can talk about their mental health and state of mind without feeling stigmatized.

## Mental fitness is a hot topic

As more people realize the importance of mental health, the mental fitness movement is rising. Online #mentalfitness hashtag has received millions of views and shares as of writing this and is steadily increasing.

Many mental fitness clubs and gyms have popped up online and in brick-and-mortar institutions. Online mental health gyms as well as mental health spas.

Companies can also benefit from mental fitness gyms. Employers can offer this perk to their employees to improve their mental health for a more productive, efficient workplace.

Nothing is a more powerful than our minds. Negative thoughts are like dark holes and they can most certainly make you feel inferior and unworthy.

This can lead to making you want to stay in bed for a whole day and still not realize the depths of the negative state you are in. That is why it is so important to rid negative thoughts as they are so bad for the body and mind. The worst part of negative thoughts is that you may sometimes know where they are originating from, but it can feel hopeless trying to face the fight of the long hard battle of fixing the root cause.

You may be in your kitchen or bedroom feeling vibrant and happy and the next thing you start to feel gloomy. Negative thinking hits you like a tsunami. You may start to only see your flaws, failures, and even your fears. Perhaps begin to believe you are a mistake and reason for all of the shortcomings.

High-stress levels are a major factor in emotional pain. When you're constantly stressed, even the slightest movement provokes you. You can end up channeling all your anger either to yourself or a second innocent party which is unfair and unjust.

Stress is a predisposing factor to emotional baggage. Stress can also cause heart failure.

Stress affects sleep rhythm. Stress distorts how we sleep and our day suffers from it. This is the reason scientists believe emotional pain manifests in the physical world.

# Mental Fitness On Steroids

My journey was indeed extreme, perhaps like mental fitness on steroids. The real bootcamp is to do what I did and keep the mental strength to stay on track day after day for the rest of your life. No, this is not the norm. However, it is possible once you turn on your mental fitness switch; you can do just about anything; and sustain.

It can be compared to physical fitness. The "norm" could be that you go to the gym every day but then eat poorly, drink too much alcohol, or get little sleep. The gym is surely helpful, but you won't be able to live up to your full potential unless you comprehend what it takes to be truly physically fit.

Mental fitness is the same. Journaling, or other efforts and activities are all wonderful; however, while these exercises are helpful, you won't be able to achieve proper mental fitness unless you understand how the mind works.

My mental fitness has been the guidance for the human mental experiences I have had and trained others to as well. I have personally become more grounded and mentally driven. You have to do more than just the individual exercises if you want to be mentally healthy which lasts and manifests.

Mental fitness is not a panacea but more so preparation.

Although improving your mental health won't suddenly solve all of your difficulties, it is a crucial first step and has a significant impact on the end outcome. Mental fitness will make one more capable of working out whatever life has around the corner.

In conclusion, you are your vessel, and I urge you to look at your entirety as something you can continue to fill. Where there are holes, fill them. "Mental fitness can be like an insurance plan" (as I read somewhere). This couldn't be truer. It helps to acknowledge all of the amazing things your mind stores and has in store, so why not also protect it?

Manufactured by Amazon.ca
Acheson, AB